GARGOURI Marwa
GARGOURI Héla

Assessment of nursing knowledge about tuberculosis

GARGOURI Marwa
GARGOURI Héla

Assessment of nursing knowledge about tuberculosis

Nursing knowledge of tuberculosis: epidemiology, modes of transmission, treatment and prevention

ScienciaScripts

Imprint
Any brand names and product names mentioned in this book are subject to trademark, brand or patent protection and are trademarks or registered trademarks of their respective holders. The use of brand names, product names, common names, trade names, product descriptions etc. even without a particular marking in this work is in no way to be construed to mean that such names may be regarded as unrestricted in respect of trademark and brand protection legislation and could thus be used by anyone.

Cover image: www.ingimage.com

This book is a translation from the original published under ISBN 978-620-6-71526-9.

Publisher:
Sciencia Scripts
is a trademark of
Dodo Books Indian Ocean Ltd. and OmniScriptum S.R.L publishing group

120 High Road, East Finchley, London, N2 9ED, United Kingdom
Str. Armeneasca 28/1, office 1, Chisinau MD-2012, Republic of Moldova, Europe
Printed at: see last page
ISBN: 978-620-7-78928-3

Copyright © GARGOURI Marwa, GARGOURI Héla
Copyright © 2024 Dodo Books Indian Ocean Ltd. and OmniScriptum S.R.L publishing group

TABLE OF CONTENTS

INTRODUCTION

It's obvious that human beings are always striving for a well-balanced state of health. However, the factors and elements that can upset this balance are enormous and can be found everywhere, even in the air we breathe. The latter is a means of transmission for many diseases, such as tuberculosis. The history of tuberculosis traces the development of knowledge about this pathology, whose existence seems as old as that of the human race, but whose aetiological unity was not established until the 19th century[1]. This infectious disease is the result of contamination by a bacterium called Koch's bacillus, discovered in Germany by Robert Koch in 1882. At the time, morbidity and mortality rates were very high, and treatment only became available with the invention of antibiotics and the BCG vaccine at the beginning of the 20th century.Despite medical advances, tuberculosis is still a public health problem in many countries around the world. In Tunisia, there has been a slight reduction in the number of cases recorded each year per 100,000 inhabitants. These results can be explained by the development of the national tuberculosis control programme. However, there are still problems with equipment and facilities, which are hampering the proper treatment of patients with tuberculosis, hence the need to re-evaluate this treatment in order to identify the factors causing these problems. In all of this, the role of the nurse is vital, as he or she is the the healthcare staff most responsible for screening, referring and caring for patients. It is therefore important that nursing knowledge is sufficiently adaptable and compatible with these tasks. The aim of our project is to assess nurses' theoretical and practical knowledge of tuberculosis in order to identify shortcomings and lack of knowledge, and to describe the difficulties encountered during treatment.

MATERIALS AND METHODS

I. Type of study :

This is a descriptive, cross-sectional study of health workers at Gabès University Hospital, aimed at assessing nurses' knowledge of tuberculosis.

II. Study environment and period :

The survey was carried out at the University Hospital of Gabès over a three-month period from February to April 2023.

The departments included in our study were the following:

- Infectious Diseases Department

- Pneumology Department

- Emergency department

III. The target population :

Our study targets all nursing staff working in the above departments.

1. Inclusion criteria :

- Staff working in the pneumology, infectious diseases and emergency departments.
- Nurses who agreed to take part in our survey and who were present at the time of the study
- Nurses of all ages and both sexes

- Nurses who work mornings, evenings and nights

2. Non-inclusion criteria :

- Staff who refused to take part in our survey

- Nurses on leave during the data collection period

- Staff working in other departments

IV. The data collection instrument :

The data was collected using a questionnaire (Appendix 1) written in French, anonymous and composed of 36 questions divided into two parts:

• Part 1: Socio-demographic and professional characteristics: gender, age, seniority in the department, the department in which they work.
• Part 2: Study of knowledge: definition of tuberculosis, formation, epidemiology, types, clinical signs, etiopathogenesis, etc.
➢ **The first dimension: theoretical knowledge :**

The questions cover all the general information about tuberculosis (definition, epidemiology, locations, clinical signs and preventive measures, etc.).

☐ A correct answer: 1 point

☐ A partially correct answer: receives 0.5 points

☐ A wrong answer: gets 0 points

The score is obtained by adding together the marks awarded for each question. It varies between 0 and 28 points. A high score indicates a good level of theoretical knowledge.

☐ A score between 0 and 9 points is considered low

☐ A score between 10 and 19 points is considered: average

☑A score between 20 and 28 points is considered high
➢ **The second dimension: practical knowledge :**

The questions in this section related to nurses' practices in the face of tuberculosis, covering compliance with universal precautions, emergency care and hospitalisation.

The score varies between 0 and 6 points, and two categories were defined:
☐ Poor practice: a score of 0 to 3.5 points

☑Good practice: a score of 4 to 6 points

V. Conduct of the study :

Our survey was carried out between 01/02/2023 and 19/04/2023 in the three departments mentioned above at the University Hospital of Gabès. Each employee spent an average of 20 minutes answering the various parts of the questionnaire.

VI. Ethical considerations :

Ethical considerations were respected throughout the data collection and analysis procedure:

• The questionnaire is strictly anonymous in order to guarantee maximum objectivity in the responses, and the confidential nature of the data is respected in accordance with the standards of the study.
• The head of department's authorisation was granted prior to data collection.
• The purpose of the study is clearly explained to study participants before data collection.

VII. Data analysis :

Once the data had been collected, the questionnaire results were processed using Excel and Word 2007 software.

VIII. Difficulties encountered :

- Some staff refused to answer the questionnaire, while others were careless in their responses.

- Some people were reluctant to respond to our questionnaire on time.

ANALYSIS OF RESULTS

A. Socio-demographic and professional characteristics :

During our study period, 60 healthcare workers were included.

1. Genre:

Our population consisted of 39 women (65%) and 21 men (35%), with a sex ratio (M/F) of 0.53 (Figure 1).

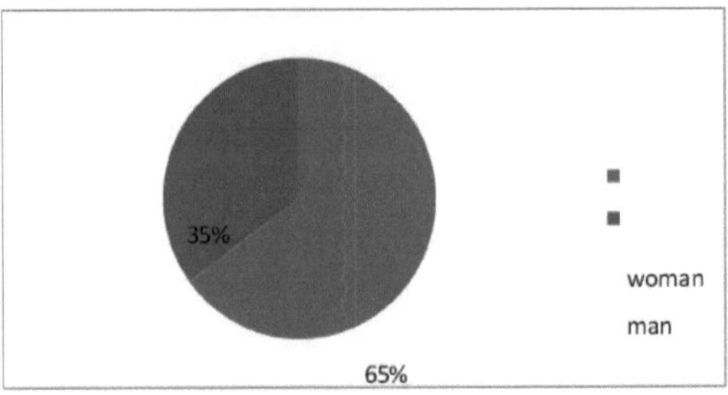

Figure 1: breakdown of nurses by gender

2. Age :

In our survey we found that the dominant age category is under 30 (42%) (Figure 2).

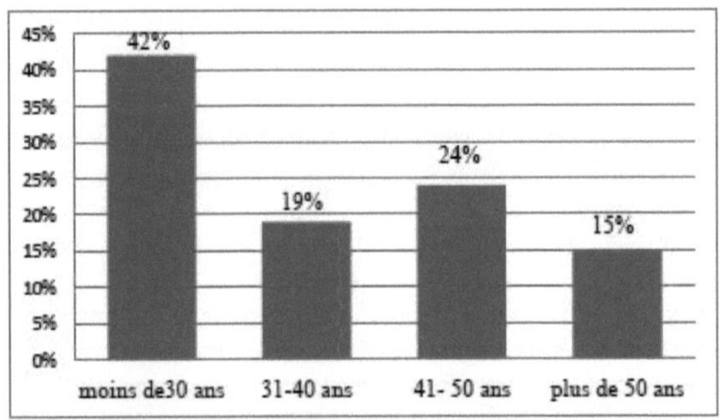

Figure 2: Breakdown of nurses by age

3. Length of service :

➤ The majority of staff surveyed have less than 5 years' professional experience (37%) (Figure 3).

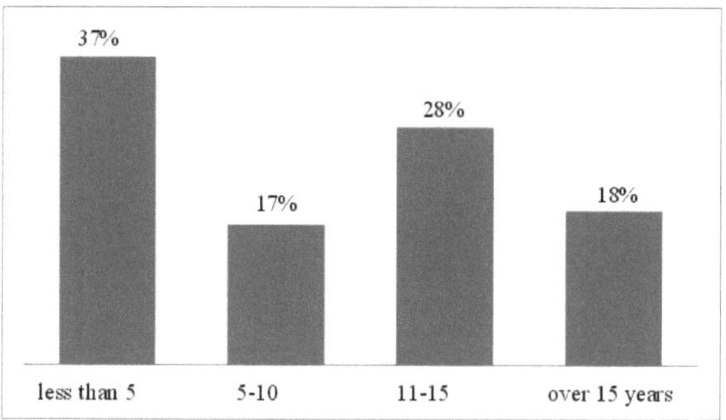

Figure 3: Breakdown of nurses by length of service in the departments

4. Work services :

We found that the number of staff questioned was almost similar in the three departments, with a slight predominance for the emergency department (43%) (Table 1).

Table 1: Breakdown of nurses by department

Employment services	Workforce	Percentage (%)
Emergencies		
	26	43
Pneumology		
	18	30
Infectious diseases		
	16	27

5. The working period :

The majority of nurses work in the morning from 7am to 1pm, with a percentage
of 43% (Figure 4).

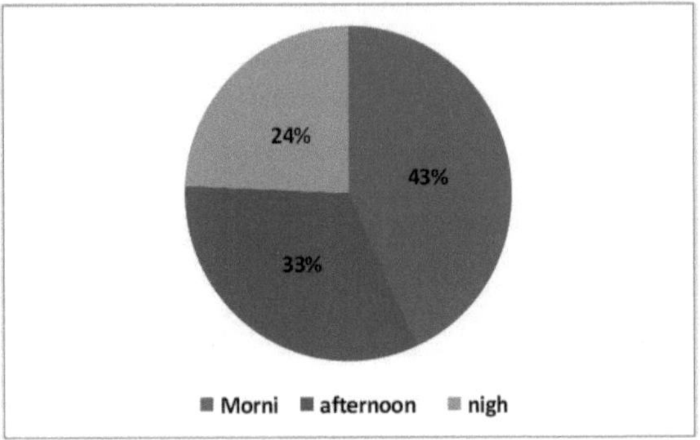

Figure 4: Breakdown of nurses by working period.

B. Study of general knowledge about tuberculosis :
I. The definition of tuberculosis :
1. Have an idea about tuberculosis:

➤ The number of nurses who had no idea about tuberculosis was 3, with a
percentage of 5% (Figure 5).

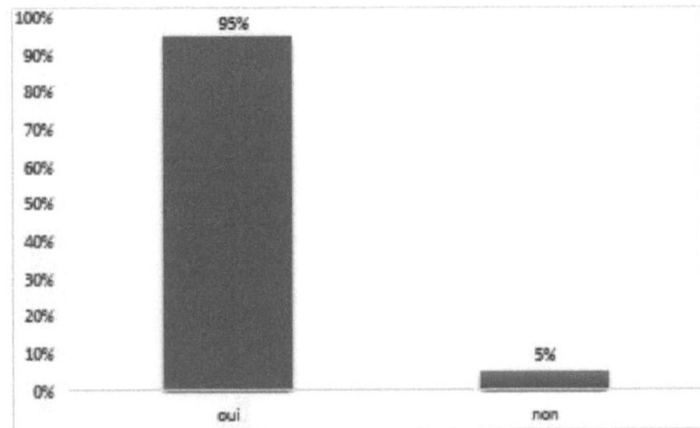

**Figure 5: Distribution of nurses according to their knowledge of the term
tuberculosis**

2. The definition of tuberculosis :

We have proposed 3 definitions of this disease:

• The first is a chronic progressive infection with a latent phase and possibly an active phase.
• The second is an infectious disease caused by a mycobacterium, Mycobacterium tuberculosis, which most often affects the lungs but can also affect other organs.
• The third is a contagious disease caused by the koch bacillus and certain external causes (malnutrition, lack of sunlight, etc.).

We found that the majority chose the second definition (Table 2).

Table 2: Distribution of nurses by definition of tuberculosis

The definition	Workforce	Percentage (%)
Is a chronic progressive infection including a latency phase and possibly an active phase	8	11
This is an infectious disease caused by a mycobacterium, Mycobacterium tubeculosis, which most often affects the lungs.	33	47
Contagious disease caused by the koch bacillus and certain external causes (malnutrition, lack of food, etc.).of sunshine)	29	42

II. Participation in a training course on tuberculosis :

Staff who took part in training courses on tuberculosis wereby 32%.

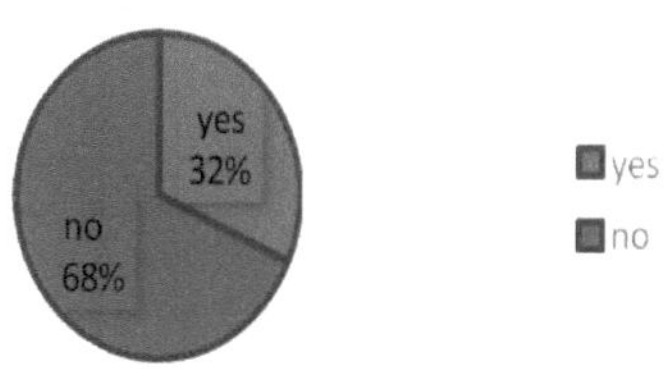

Figure 6 :Distribution ofnurses according to participation in training on tuberculosis

III. The epidemiology of tuberculosis :

1. The number of cases reported in 2021 in Tunisia :

According to our results, the majority of nurses chose the response "36 new cases of tuberculosis per 100,000 inhabitants" (35%) (Figure 7).

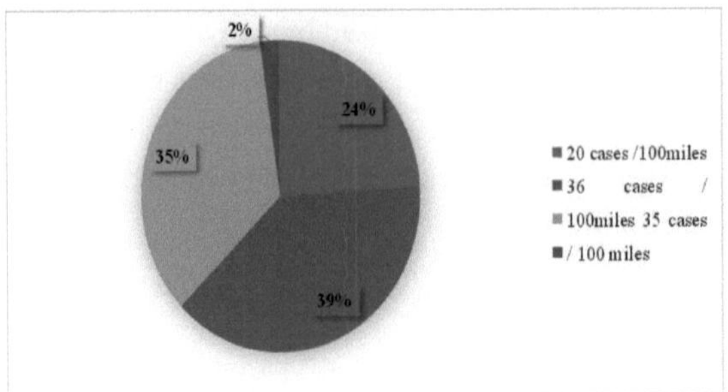

Figure 7: Distribution of nurses according to newly reported cases of tuberculosis in 2021.

2. The incidence of tuberculosis in the Gabès region :

Half of our sample stated that the incidence of tuberculosis in the Gabès region is close to the national average (57%) (Table 3).

Table 3: Incidence of tuberculosis in the Gabès region

The impact is :	The workforce	The percentage(%)
Significantly lower than average national	12	20
Close to the average national	34	57
Above average national	14	23

IV. The different types of tuberculosis :

1. The most common tuberculosis sites:

According to our results, the lung and lymph node types represent the dominant locations, with percentages of 29% and 28% respectively (Figure 10).

Table 4: Distribution of nurses according to the most common tuberculosis sites encountered

Types of tuberculosis	The workforce	The percentage (%)
Pulmonary	43	29
Ganglion	41	28
Peritoneal	28	19
Bone	17	11
Neuromeningeal	11	7
Multiple locations	7	5
Other	2	1
Skin	0	0

2. Adenopathies in lymph node tuberculosis :

For the entire population surveyed, adenopathies were located in the cervical and mediastinal regions, with percentages of 58% and 25% respectively (Figure 8).

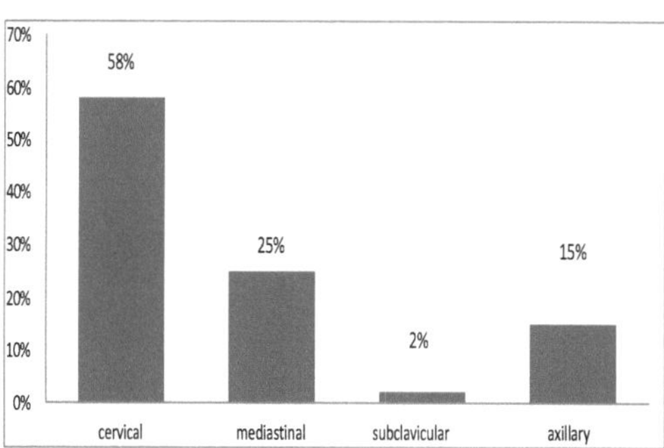

Figure 8: Distribution of nurses according to the most frequent location of adenopathies in lymph node tuberculosis

3. Organs affected by peritoneal tuberculosis :

According to our study, the parietal and visceral peritoneum (28%) and the intestinal tract (25%) are the peritoneal organs most affected by tuberculosis, while the spleen and genital organs (10%) are in the minority (Figure 5).

Table 5: Distribution of nurses according to organs affected by peritoneal tuberculosis

Organs affected	The workforce	Percentage (%)
Parietal and visceral peritoneum	30	28
Intestinal tract	26	25
The liver	16	15
The omentum	13	12
Spleen	11	10
The genitals	11	10

V. Clinical signs of tuberculosis :

Cough, fever and weight loss were the clinical signs most frequently selected by nurses in our study population, followed by fatigue and haemoptysis (Figure 6).

Table 6: Distribution of nurses according to clinical signs of tuberculosis

The symptoms	The workforce	Percentage (%)
Persistent cough for more than 2 weeks	37	12
Weight loss	37	12
Fever	37	12
Fatigue	36	11
Haemoptysis	31	10
Anorexia	27	9
Night sweats	27	9
Adenopathies	23	8
Infectious syndrome	17	6
Vomiting	15	5
Joint pain	13	4
Diarrhoea	7	2

VI. Etiopathogenesis :

1. Class of germ responsible for tuberculosis :

According to the survey results, 90% of tuberculosis cases are bacterial (Figure 9).

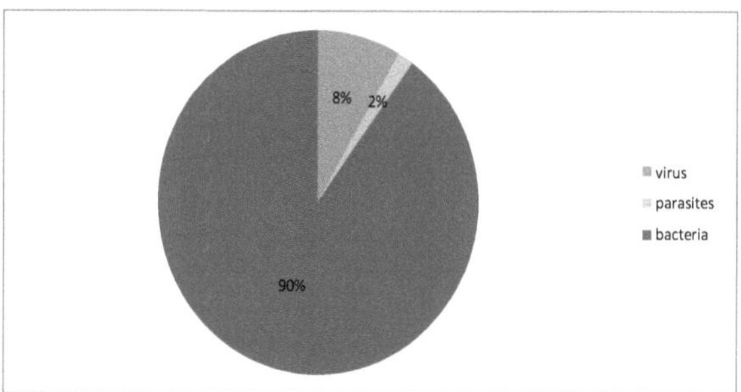

Figure 9: Distribution of nurses by class of germ responsible for tuberculosis

2. The bacterium that causes tuberculosis :

The results of the research show that koch's bacilli are the bacteria responsible for tuberculosis (100%) (Figure 10).

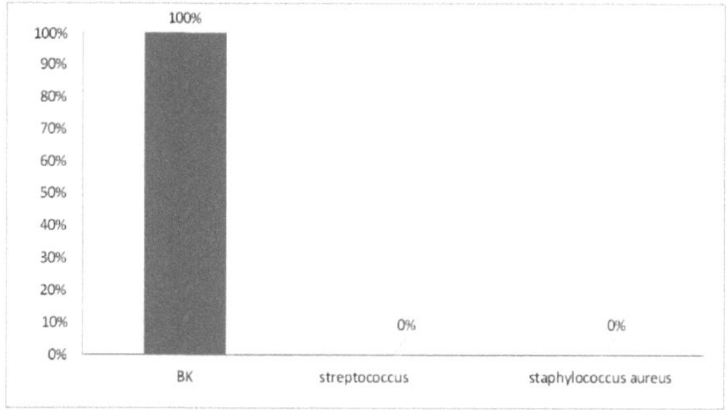

Figure 10: Distribution of nurses according to the bacterium causing tuberculosis

1. Reservoirs of tuberculosis :

The majority of nurses replied that there are other reservoirs of tuberculosis other than humans (82%) (figure11).

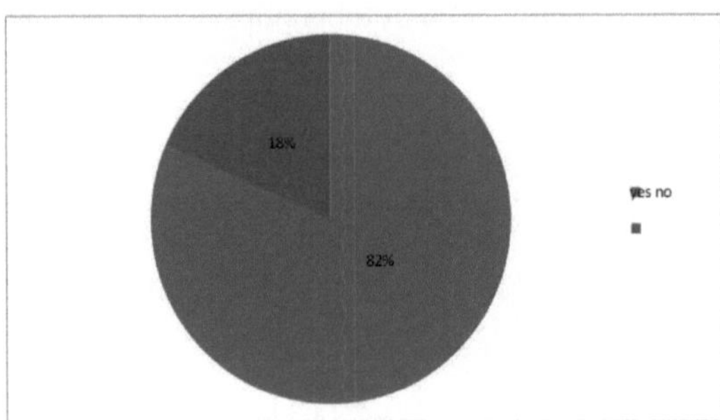

Figure 11: Breakdown of nurses by reservoir in the tuberculosis

2. Modes of transmission of tuberculosis :

In our study, we found that, according to the nurses, tuberculosis is mainly transmitted by air (56%) (Figure 12).

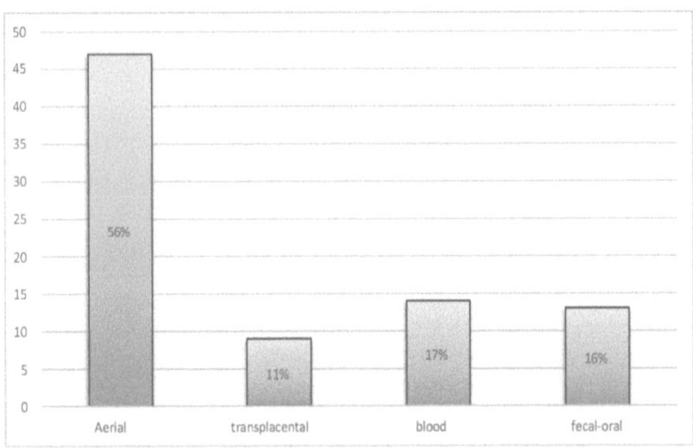

Figure 12: Distribution of nurses according to modes of transmission of tuberculosis.

1. Transmission of pulmonary tuberculosis :

For our population, transmission of pulmonary tuberculosis is mainly by air (87%) (figure13).

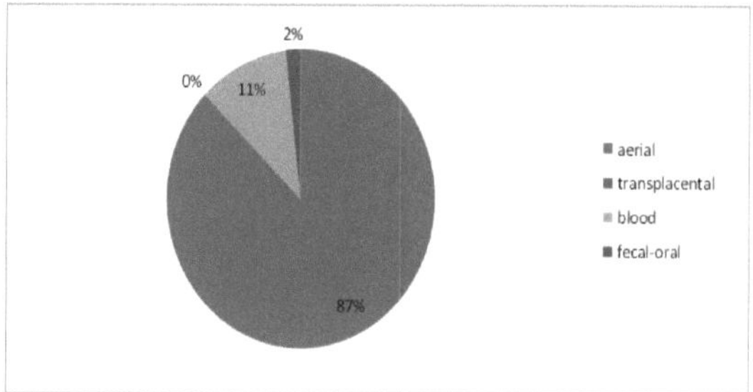

Figure 13: Distribution of nurses according to transmission of pulmonary tuberculosis

2. The mode of dissemination of extra pulmonary tuberculosis :

According to the results of our survey, the majority of nurses replied that extra pulmonary tuberculosis is usually due to haematogenous dissemination of pulmonary tuberculosis (figure 14).

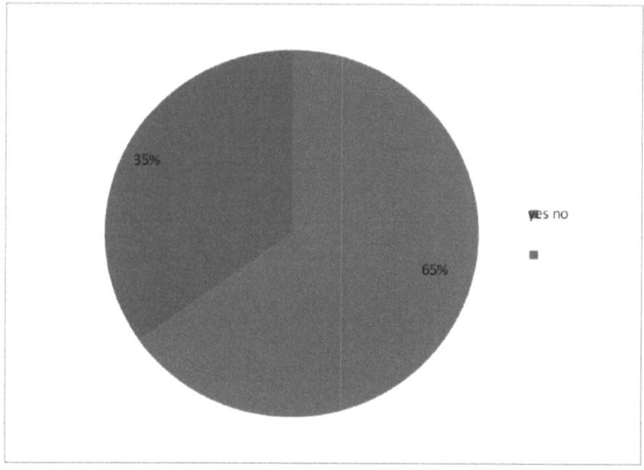

Figure 14: Distribution of nurses according to the spread of pulmonary tuberculosis

6. Stages of tuberculosis :

The percentages of staff corresponding to each proposal were very close. According to our nurses, the first phase was latent infection (39%), the second phase was primary infection (21%) and the final phase was active infection in 29% of cases (Figure 15).

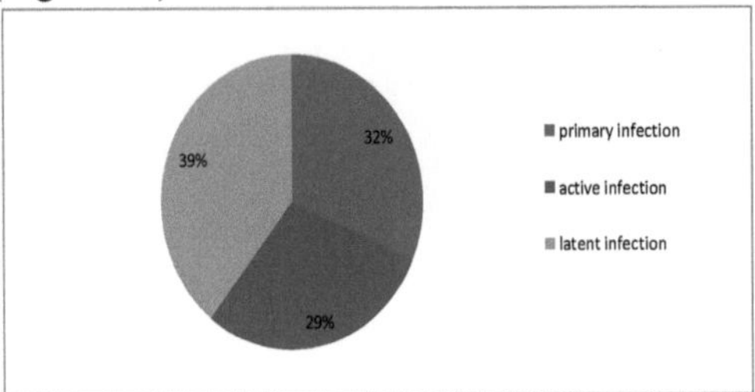

Figure 15: Distribution of nurses by stage of tuberculosis.

7. Risk factors for tuberculosis :

For our population, lack of BCG vaccination and immune deficiency are the main risk factors for tuberculosis, with percentages of 20% and 16% respectively (table 7).

Table 7: Distribution of nurses according to tuberculosis risk factors.

Risk factors	Workforce	Percentage (%)
Promiscuity	13	7
Malnutrition	26	13
Children under 5 years of age	6	3
Elderly people	16	8
Diabetes	21	11
Immune deficiency	31	16
Unfavourable socio-economic conditions	25	13
Vitamin D deficiency	3	1
No BCG vaccination	40	20
Drug and tobacco use	16	8

VI. Screening tests for tuberculosis :

For our population, sputum BK and TST are the main tests used to detect tuberculosis, with percentages of 35% and 29% respectively (Figure 16).

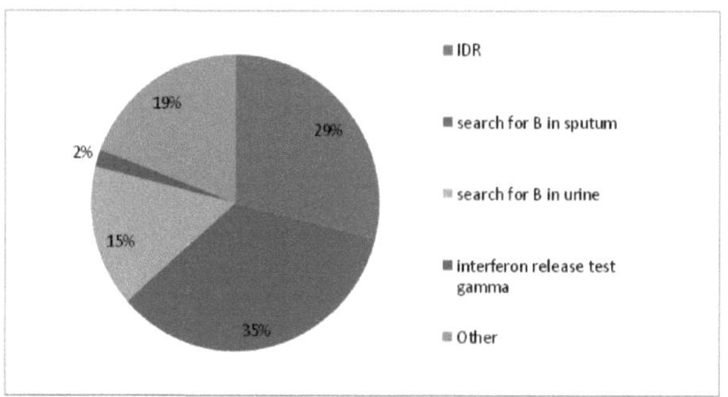

Figure 16: Distribution of nurses according to tuberculosis screening tests

Nurses suggested other screening tests such as chest X-rays (11%) and chest scans (Table 8).

Table 8: Other examinations proposed by nurses.

Other	Percentage (%)
Chest X-ray	11%
Chest scan	4%
Adenopathy biopsy	2%
Skin test	1%
Acetylation test	1%

VII. Potential complications of tuberculosis :

For our population, respiratory failure (21%) and extension to other sites (19%) are the potential complications of tuberculosis (table 9).

Complications	workforce	Percentage (%)
The caves	18	12
Respiratory failure	32	21
Arteritis and osteitis	21	14
Pulmonary embolism	17	11
Occlusion	2	1
Fistula	10	7
Superinfection	22	15
Extension to other locations	29	19

Table 9: Distribution of nurses according to potential complications of tuberculosis

VIII. Treatment and management of tuberculosis :

1. Distribution of nurses according to the therapeutic class used in the treatment of tuberculosis :

The majority of nurses surveyed (63%) indicated that anti-tuberculosis drugs are the main treatment for tuberculosis (Figure 17).

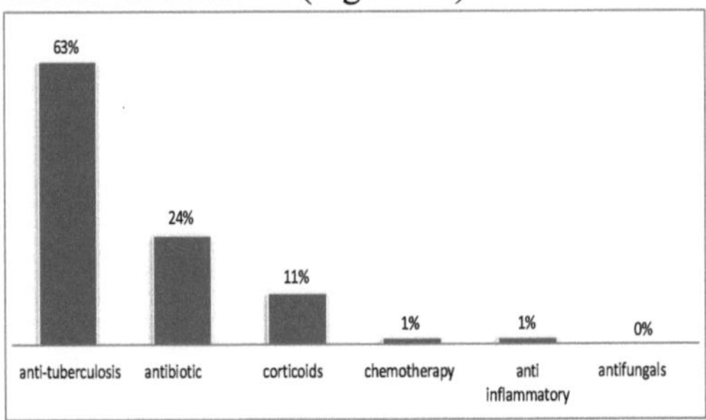

Figure 17: Distribution of nurses according to the therapeutic class used to treat tuberculosis.

2. The cost of treating tuberculosis :

According to our recent study, 97% of the population surveyed responded that tuberculosis treatment is free (Figure 18).

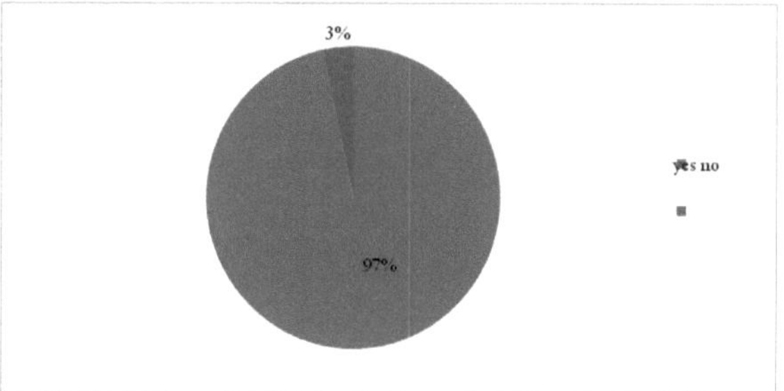

Figure 18: Distribution of nurses according to whether tuberculosis treatment is free of charge

IX. Preventive measures :

1. BCG vaccine :

Most nurses replied that all newborns should be vaccinated against tuberculosis (33%) (Table 10).

Table 10: Distribution of nurses by BCG vaccination

The proposals :	The workforce	Percentages (%)
P1: a live attenuated vaccine	30	26
P2: the vial of vaccine contains at least 10 doses.	13	11
P3: the vaccine is given as a strict intradermal injection	29	25
P4: all newborn babies should be vaccinated	38	33
P5: BCG is indicated for pregnant women and immunocompromised patients	5	5

2. Isolation :

The majority of nurses (68%) did not see the need for isolation in all types of tuberculosis (Figure 19).

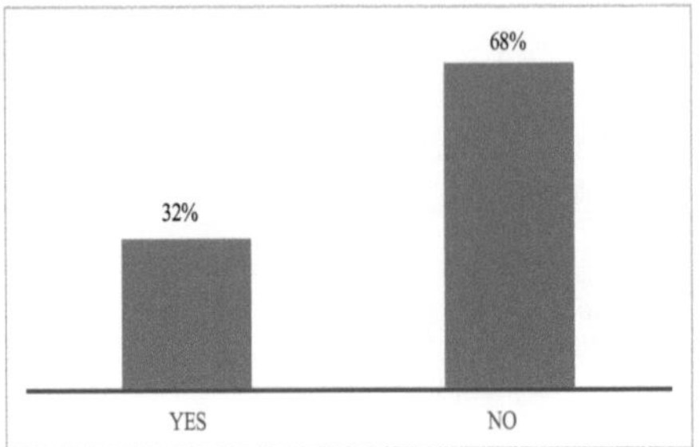

Figure 19: Distribution of nurses according to the indication for isolation in cases of tuberculosis

I. Isolation in the case of pulmonary tuberculosis :

All the nurses stressed the importance and necessity of isolation in cases of pulmonary tuberculosis (figure 20).

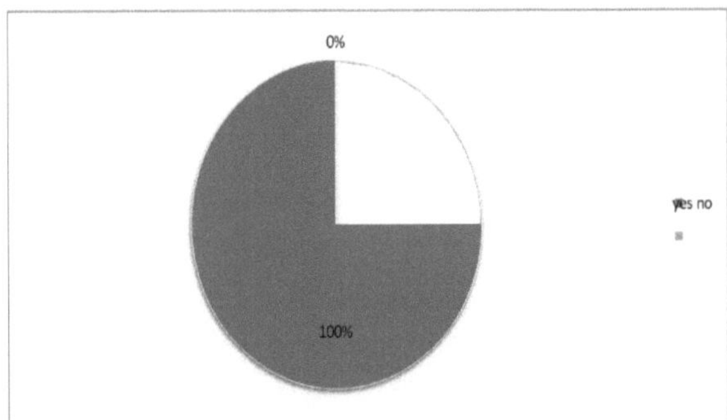

Figure 20: Distribution of nurses according to the need for isolation in cases of pulmonary tuberculosis.

II. Wearing bibs:

We found that 89% of nurses wore bibs when caring for a patient with tuberculosis (Figure 21).

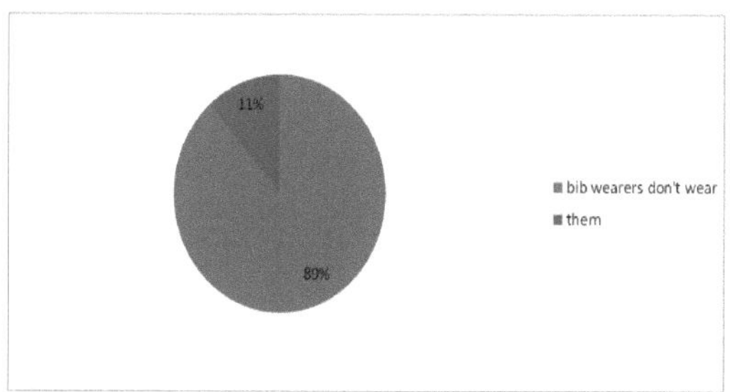

Figure 21: Distribution of nurses by wearing of bibs.

III. Declaring tuberculosis :

According to the nurses questioned, tuberculosis is a notifiable disease, with a percentage of 100%. (Figure 22)

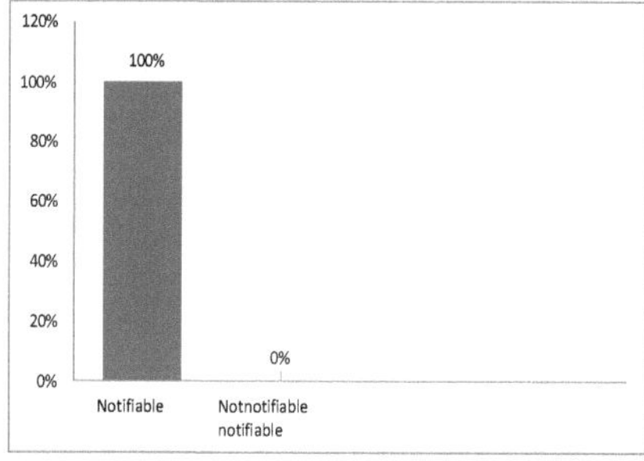

Figure 22: Distribution of nurses according to tuberculosis notification.

IV. Authorities involved in the declaration :

The majority of participants in our study chose to report to the regional health authority (60%) (Figure 23).

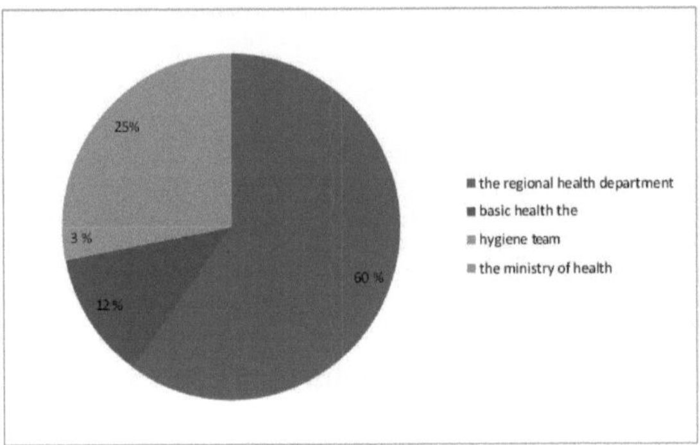

Figure 23: Distribution of nurses by reporting authority.

V. The need for a health survey of those close to a patient :

We noted that most of the subjects interviewed indicated that the survey was necessary for prevention, in order to detect new cases (56%) (Figure 24).

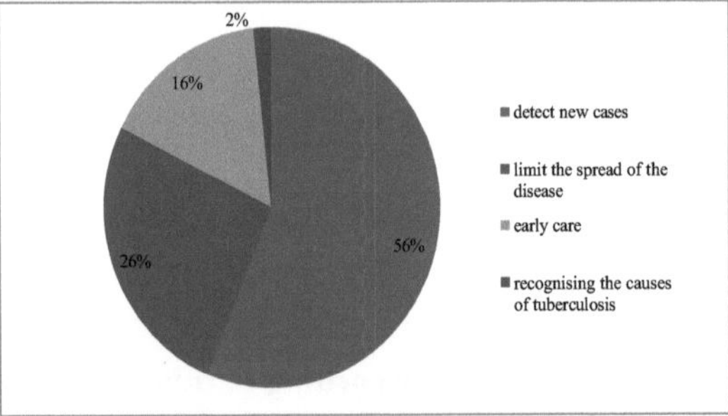

Figure 24: Distribution of nurses according to the need for a health survey of a patient's family and friends.

VI.Objectives of the national tuberculosis control programme :

> Analysis of the data collected revealed that the majority of nurses indicated that the objectives of the national tuberculosis control programme were to reduce morbidity and mortality (61%) (Table 11).

Table 11: Objectives of the national tuberculosis control programme

Objective	Number Percentage
Tuberculosis will no longer be a public health problem by 2050	14 23%
Incidence falls below 1 per million population	10 16%
Reducing morbidity and mortality	37 61%

Theoretical knowledge score :

In our survey, it follows from the above that the general level of theoretical knowledge about tuberculosis is average (16.5/28), and this may be related to the fact that most of the nurses questioned had not taken part in previous training courses.

Table 12: Assessment of theoretical knowledge

The number of points	
The definition of tuberculosis	0.5/2
Training on tuberculosis	0/1
Epidemiology	0.5/2
Types of tuberculosis	2/3
Clinical signs	1/1
Etiopathology	5.5/8
Screening tests	0.5/1
Complications	0.5/1
Treatments	1 / 2
Preventive measures	5/7
Total points	16,5/28

IX. The nursing role in the management of tuberculosis :

1. Previous management of patients with tuberculosis, regardless of location

The results obtained for this question showed that 87% of the population studied managed patients with tuberculosis (Figure 25).

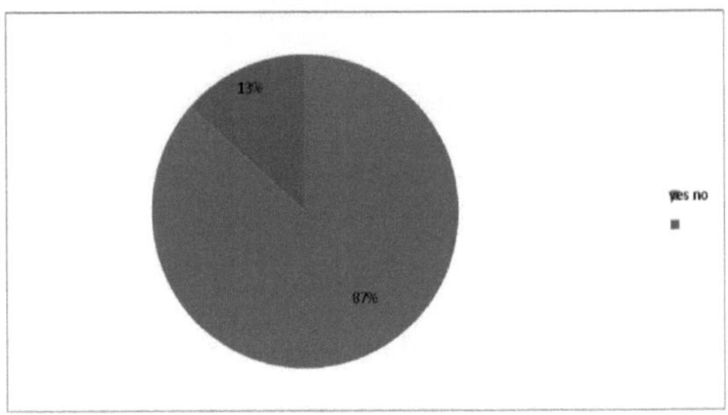

Figure 25: Distribution of nurses according to previous tuberculosis treatment

✓ **Location of tuberculosis :**

According to our results, we found that pulmonary tuberculosis was the location most frequently encountered (52%) (Figure 26).

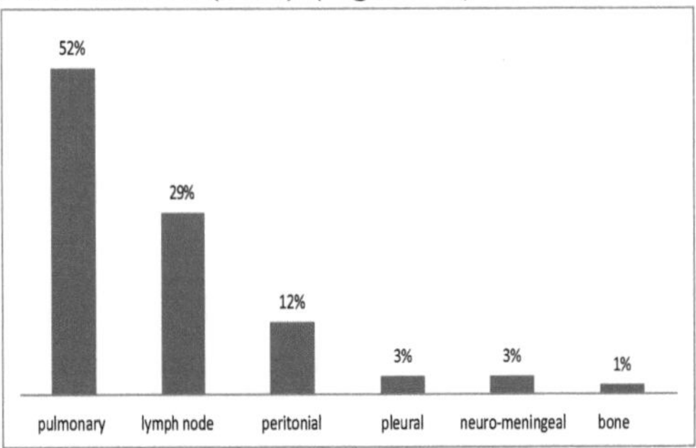

Figure 26: Distribution of nurses by location of tuberculosis in patients under their care.

✓ **ACTION TO BE TAKEN :**

- The nurse's response to a patient with tuberculosis in an emergency :

In our survey, we noted that screening examinations were chosen by 54% of participants as the most appropriate way of dealing with tuberculosis in an emergency, and that reporting and isolating patients was cited by 33% of healthcare workers. (Table 13)

Table 13: Distribution of nurses according to emergency procedures

	Workforce	Percentage
undergo a screening test on medical prescription	26	44%
peripheral venous access	16	27%
oxygen therapy	12	19%
monitoring vital parameters	6	10%

-

The conduct of nurses during hospitalisation in the two pneumology and infectious diseases departments when faced with a tuberculosis patient:

Analysis of the data collected revealed that 47% of nurses insisted on administering anti-tuberculosis treatments and 23% suggested monitoring the general state of health. (Table 14).

Table 14: Distribution of nurses according to the Instructions for Use during hospitalisation in the two pulmonology and infectious diseases departments

Workforce		Percentage
administration of anti-tuberculosis treatments	35	47%
general condition monitoring	17	23%
screening tests	11	14%
good patient compliance during treatment	7	10%
isolation	5	6%

2. Nurses' level of satisfaction with tuberculosis care :

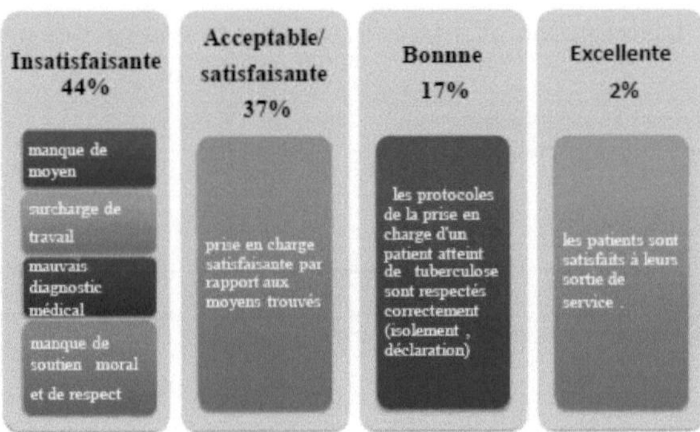

Figure 27: Assessment of nurses' satisfaction with tuberculosis care.

3. Nurses' proposals for better tuberculosis care :

Nurses emphasised two key aspects for improving tuberculosis management: providing the hospital with all the equipment needed to carry out complementary examinations and screening (39%) and providing health education (28%). (Table 15).

Table 15: Proposals for better care.

Proposals for better care	Workforce	Percentage (%)
Equipping the hospital with all the equipment needed for complementary examinations and screening	23	39
Health education	17	28
Comply with the tuberculosis control protocol	7	12
Staff training	5	8
Good nutrition for patients	5	8
Moral support	3	5

Practice score for tuberculosis :

Our survey showed that nurses had good practices in dealing with tuberculosis
(the score was 4/6). (Table 16).

Table 16: Score of tuberculosis practices.

The number of points	
What to do in an emergency	1 / 2
What to do during hospitalisation	1,5/2
Assessment of nursing care	0,5/1
Nurses' proposals	1/1
Total score	4/6

DISCUSSION

A. Characteristics socio-demographic and occupation :

Our study involved 60 nurses, 65% of whom were women. In contrast, a study carried out in Abidjan to assess the knowledge and attitudes of nurses involved in the management of TB/HIV co-infection showed a predominance of men [2].

✤ This difference is explained by the fact that the number of nurses in Tunisia is greater than that of male nurses, in line with the feminisation of the population. 36% of nurses had less than 5 years' experience and 42% were aged under 30. In contrast, the results of the previous study showed that the average age of nursing staff was 40.9 years and the average length of service was 8 years [2].The prepared questionnaire was distributed in the respiratory (30%), emergency (43%) and infectious diseases (27%) departments.

✤ These departments were chosen because patients with tuberculosis might be present.

B. Study of knowledge general a about of tuberculosis :
I. Definition of tuberculosis :

According to the national guide to the management of tuberculosis developed by the Ministry of Health (2018), tuberculosis is defined as an infectious disease caused by bacteria of the mycobacterium complex (M) tuberculosis, and can be classified as primary tuberculosis or post-primary (secondary) tuberculosis. [3]

In this case, 47% of participants indicated that tuberculosis is an infectious disease caused by a mycobacterium, Mycobacterium tuberculosis, which most often affects the lungs. The majority (89%) are unaware that tuberculosis is a chronic, progressive infection comprising a latent stage and an active stage.

II. Training on tuberculosis :

Dr Carrie Tudor, ICN TB Project Director (2019), said that continuing education for nurses on the prevention, modes of transmission, primary care and treatment of TB disease are key to improving patient care. Nurses are on the front line, every day, throughout the world. They play an essential role in better screening and detecting cases, providing patients with the appropriate treatment, monitoring patients and improving quality of life. [4]

In this context, only 32% of the nurses surveyed had taken part in training courses during their studies and in the course of their work.

↳ This may be due to a failure to recognise the importance of updating their knowledge of tuberculosis.

III. Epidemiology :

According to the World Health Organisation (WHO, 2023), the number of cases reported in Tunisia in 2021 will be 36 new cases/100,000 inhabitants. This figure is relatively low compared with South Africa, where there are 513 new cases per 100,000 inhabitants, and neighbouring countries (54 cases per 100,000 inhabitants in Algeria, 59 cases per 100,000 inhabitants in Libya and 94 cases per 100,000 inhabitants in Morocco). [5]

In this sense, 36 new cases/100miles is the proposal most chosen by the participants in our survey (35%). According to our results, almost half of our staff believe that the incidence of tuberculosis in the Gabès region is close to the national average (57%). However, according to the Gabès Regional Health Department, the incidence of tuberculosis is higher than the national average (140 cases in 2022).

IV. The different types of tuberculosis:

The results of our survey show that pulmonary tuberculosis (29%) and lymph node tuberculosis (28%) are the two most frequently reported localisations, followed by peritoneal tuberculosis (19%). We found that only 7% of nurses were aware of neuromeningeal tuberculosis, while none of our nurses mentioned cutaneous tuberculosis. A retrospective study including 100 patients treated for tuberculosis between January 2018 and June 2021 at the Pneumology Department of Jendouba Hospital showed that pulmonary tuberculosis is by far the most common (75%), followed by pleural tuberculosis (14%) and lymph node tuberculosis (13%). In addition, other rarer localizations were found such as thoracic parietal localization (2 cases), cerebral meningeal (2 cases), mammary (1 case) and cutaneous (1 case). [6]

↳ We noted that the results of this study carried out in Jendouba converge with our results. Thus, the rarely encountered locations (neuro-meningeal, mammary and cutaneous tuberculosis) are the same types known least frequently by the nurses participating in our survey.Lymph node tuberculosis is characterised by the appearance of several adenopathies, often palpable in the human body. 58%

of the personnel questioned replied that the cervical location is the most frequent, followed by the mediastinal location with a percentage of 25%, then the axillary location (15%) and the lymph node (15%). finally subclavicular (2%). Similarly, in a retrospective study carried out in the Sfax infectious diseases department on 50 patients with lymph node tuberculosis, adenopathies were mainly cervical (75%), followed by mediastinal (21%), supra-clavicular (9.4%) and axillary (6.3%) [7]. The results of a study carried out at the Marrakech tuberculosis centre showed that adenopathy was cervical in 95% of cases, mediastinal in 5.1%, abdominal in 3.7%, axillary in 2.8% and inguinal in 0.3%. [8] The majority of nurses chose the two most frequently encountered locations. We can therefore conclude that their knowledge is limited to the locations most frequently encountered in their work, and that they do not carry out in-depth research into the rarer ones. According to our results, the majority of staff (28%) stated that the organs that can be affected in cases of peritoneal tuberculosis are the parietal and visceral peritoneum, 25% the intestinal tract, 15% the liver, 12% the omentum and 10% the spleen and genitals. A survey carried out in the general surgery department at Marrakech Military Hospital showed the organs affected during abdominal tuberculosis. The areas most affected were the small intestine (44%), the caecum (35%) and the ileo-caecum (16%). Isolated involvement of the colon is rare, and is estimated at between The other abdominal sites involved lymph nodes, the peritoneum, the liver and the spleen. [9]

V. Clinical signs of tuberculosis :

According to the nurses' responses, the symptoms characterising this disease are very similar in percentage: fever, persistent cough lasting more than 2 weeks and weight loss (12%), fatigue (11%), haemoptysis (10%), night sweats, anorexia (9%) and adenopathy (8%). A study carried out in Côte d'Ivoire by researchers at Bouake University found that the clinical signs most suggestive of tuberculosis were: prolonged cough (87.6%), blood in the sputum (40.6%), weight loss (32.7%) and chest pain (13.9%), while the other symptoms were less common [10]. In both studies, most of the respondents mentioned tuberculosis in relation to the three main clinical signs: prolonged cough, weight loss and haemoptysis, which explains why the symptoms of tuberculosis are obvious and known by most of the staff, whatever their region or level of education.

VI. Etiopathogenesis :

According to our nurses, tuberculosis is a bacterial disease in 90% of cases. However, some believe that it was a viral and parasitic disease in 8% and 2% respectively.

↳ Although a small percentage of participants (10%) answered this question incorrectly, we do not expect them to do so, especially as they deal with many cases of tuberculosis on a daily basis.

All of the nurses thought that the germ responsible for the disease was the Mycobacterium tuberculosis hominis 100%. According to the results of our study, 82% of the population believed that humans are not the only reservoir of tuberculosis, but also cattle. In the recent literature, the term tuberculosis covers disease caused by Mycobacterium tuberculosis (of which humans are the main reservoir), but also similar disease caused by the closely related mycobacteria M. bovis, M. africanum and M. microti [11].

According to our nurses, transmission of pulmonary tuberculosis is mainly by air (87%), and the other localisations of tuberculosis are essentially due to haematogenous dissemination of pulmonary tuberculosis (65%). Similarly, a study carried out at the University of Bamako shows that contamination occurs via the airborne route in the majority of cases (97%). However, the blood-borne, mucocutaneous and digestive routes (consumption of milk contaminated with M.bovis) may also occur [12].

M.tuberculosis bacilli initially cause a primary infection, a small percentage of which eventually progress to clinical disease of varying severity. However, most (around 95%) primary infections are asymptomatic.A percentage of primary infections disappear spontaneously, but the majority are followed by a latent phase. A variable varies(5 à   10%) of infections latent infections are reactivate later with the appearance of the symptoms of the disease. [11] The disease progresses through three stages classified by most nurses in chronological order: latent infection, primary infection and then active infection.With regard to risk factors for tuberculosis, 20% of participants felt that the lack of BCG vaccination was the main cause of contamination by this disease. Also, 16% of staff were in favour of the immune deficiency, 13% for unfavourable socio-economic conditions and malnutrition and 11% for diabetes and promiscuity 7%. Similarly, The risk factors found in a retrospective study including cases of tuberculosis in the pneumology department of the Mohamed VI University

Hospital in Marrakech (2017, 2019) were: Low socioeconomic level (70.3%), promiscuity (20.3%), lack of vaccination (5%), recent tuberculosis contagion (31.9%), smoking (31.2%), cannabism (10%), kif consumption (14.5%), alcoholism (6.5%), comorbidities such as diabetes (8.7%), HTA (8%) and progressive neoplasia (3.2%). [13]

✎ We found that nurses' knowledge of the risk factors for tuberculosis is almost the same, but with some differences in terms of percentage. This can be explained by a number of factors, such as age, gender, occupational and environmental exposure, place of residence and access to healthcare.

VII. Screening test :

The nurses' responses concerning the screening tests carried out in cases of suspected tuberculosis were 29% for the TST, 35% for the BK test in sputum, 17% for the BK test in urine, 2% for the gamma interferon release test and 20% for other investigations (chest X-ray, skin test, biopsy, acetylation test).

According to a study carried out in Belgium by the Fonds des Affections Respiratoires asbl (2023), various diagnostic tools are available to detect tuberculosis: the tuberculin skin test, also known as the intradermal reaction, IGRA tests, which are more expensive blood tests that offer an alternative to the TST, and chest X-rays. And whatever the suspected location of the tuberculosis, confirmation of the diagnosis of tuberculosis disease involves bacteriological tests. For pulmonary tuberculosis, BKs are detected in morning sputum (or in secretions obtained after bronchoscopy or gastric tubing in children). The sputum is examined under a microscope and cultured. [14]

✎ In our study, the majority of participants replied that the TST and the sputum BK test were the two essential screening tests, probably because these are the tests available at the University Hospital of Gabes.

VIII. Complications:

Of the healthcare professionals participating in our study, 21% thought that respiratory failure was the main complication, while 19% chose extension to other locations. Among our nurses, 15% mentioned the possibility of superinfection and 14% referred to arteritis and osteitis. A study conducted by Gueza, in 2018 in Algeria from the records of patients hospitalised for 2 years (2015-2016). The main complications observed were: superinfection (49%), abscess (23%), pneumothorax (11%), aspergillary graft (07%), neoplastic graft (09%), haemoptysis (48%), pulmonary embolism (08%) and tuberculosis reactivation in 4 cases. 33% of patients developed chronic respiratory failure, 03 patients underwent surgery and unfortunately we recorded 03 deaths. [15]

↳ It appears that both studies had similar complications, although the percentages were different. It is therefore important for healthcare professionals to take these complications into account and implement prevention and treatment measures to improve patient health and clinical outcomes. It is illegitimate to emphasise that prevention is always preferable to treatment, so the Health professionals should also put in place measures to prevent these complications, particularly in high-risk patients.

IX. Tuberculosis treatments :

During our study, nurses were asked about the treatments used to treat tuberculosis. The responses were as follows: 63% chose anti-tuberculosis drugs (63%), followed by antibiotics (24%), corticoids and anti-inflammatories (11%) and chemotherapy (1%). The difference in percentage between the first two propositions (63% and 24%) shows that nurses do not know that anti-tuberculosis drugs are antibiotics. A study conducted at the Institut Pasteur in 2021 shows that a combination of antibiotics is used to treat tuberculosis patients and that this treatment must be followed up for at least 6 months (and up to two years in the case of multi-resistant strains). [16]

In addition, to assess whether adjuvant corticosteroid therapy reduces mortality and accelerates clinical or microbiological recovery in people with pulmonary TB, studies indexed between 1966 and May 2014 searching the Cochrane Infectious Diseases Group Trials Register showed that Adjuvant corticosteroid therapy is unlikely to provide significant benefits for peoplewith pulmonary tuberculosis. The short-term clinical benefits we found do not appear to be sustained over the long term. [17]

In addition, a number of studies were carried out by Dr Carl Nathanr et all to test the action of anti-inflammatory drugs on BK. They found that oxyphenbutazone (an anti-inflammatory) could kill the bacteria. But it was not enough to have determined the molecule's efficacy: it still had to be tested on humans as part of an action against tuberculosis. [18] In short, tuberculosis is essentially treated by a combination of anti-tuberculosis antibiotics, as most of our nurses have

indicated (isoniazid, rifampicin, pyrazinamide, ethambutol and/or streptomycin). As far as other molecules are concerned, such as anti-inflammatory drugs and corticosteroids, their action on tuberculosis has not yet been well proven. The majority of our nurses (97%) say that tuberculosis treatments are made available to patients free of charge. The National Tuberculosis Control Programme provides free treatment for all tuberculosis patients, regardless of their location, geographical origin or source (public or private). Each patient must have a record of
A "tuberculosis patient" who has access to this free service. [19]

☙ Making free treatment available to all sufferers is an incentive for sufferers to seek treatment. As a result, we limit morbidity and mortality and the transmission of the disease. Nurses must therefore be aware of this right if they are to provide better care.

X. Preventive measures :

Regarding the BCG vaccine, 30% of nurses insisted that all newborn babies should be vaccinated, and 95% were against vaccinating pregnant women and immunocompromised patients. With regard to the characteristics of the vaccine, it is estimated that 26% of participants said that it consists of live attenuated bacilli. 11% of staff thought that the vial contained at least 10 doses and that it was to be given by strict intradermal injection (25%). According to national guidelines for the fight against tuberculosis, the BCG vaccine is recommended for all newborn babies. BCG is a live attenuated vaccine administered intradermally. The recommended dose is 0.05 ml for newborns and infants under the age of three months, and 0.1 ml for other children. However, it is contraindicated for children with immunodeficiency, as it can cause serious health problems for them. [20]

☙ We found that a minority of healthcare workers were aware that BCG vaccination is recommended for newborns and that it is administered intradermally. This can be explained by the fact that our survey was not carried out in the departments concerned with vaccination (basic health centre, maternity and neonatology departments), as knowledge and skills may vary according to their training, experience and specific area of work.

In addition, more than half (68%) of the staff questioned insisted on isolating patients with tuberculosis, whatever the location. However, they all agreed

(100%) that patients with pulmonary tuberculosis must be isolated and only come into contact with health care staff wearing bibs. Contradictorily, only 88% of nurses insisted on wearing masks. A study carried out in Belgium in 2013 showed that in cases of tuberculosis, isolation is recommended for patients with active and contagious forms of the disease. Wearing a respiratory mask is also recommended for these patients. Wearing a respiratory mask is also recommended for patients with active tuberculosis and for healthcare staff who are in direct contact with them. [21]

✎ In the case of tuberculosis, isolation and the wearing of masks are very important to prevent transmission of the disease to other people, particularly healthcare professionals. It is encouraging to see that all the staff surveyed agree on the need to isolate patients with pulmonary tuberculosis, as this is essential to prevent the spread of the disease. However, it is worrying that only 88% of nurses insist on wearing masks, as this can endanger their own health as well as that of other patients and medical and paramedical staff. It is important that all healthcare workers are aware of the importance of wearing masks as a matter of principle, as well as the other precautions needed to prevent the transmission of tuberculosis.

Analysis of the data collected revealed that all the participants confirmed that tuberculosis is a notifiable disease (100%), and that the nurses questioned reported the disease to the regional health directorate (60%), the basic health centre (12%), the hygiene team (3%) and the Ministry of Health (25%). After reporting the disease, healthcare workers emphasised the need to carry out a health survey of the people around them in order to detect new cases (58%), limit the spread of the disease (26%), treat patients early (16%) and recognise the causes of tuberculosis (2%). Reporting cases of tuberculosis is integrated into the diseases system Notifiable communicable diseases (MDO) (Law 07/12 of 12 February 2007 on communicable diseases). The information is sent using a form in duplicate, one of which is sent to the regional level (regional basic healthcare service via the health district team) and the second to the central level (DSSB). The information circuit involves health structures at 3 levels: peripheral (CSB and health district), regional (regional public health service within the regional public health directorate) and national (Directorate of Basic Health Care). [22]

✎ Nurses obviously need to be aware that tuberculosis is a notifiable disease, to ensure that as many cases as possible are detected and reported to the health authorities. With regard to the possible proposals for the objectives of the national tuberculosis control programme, the participants in our study chose the proposals with very variable percentages. The majority (61%) chose to reduce morbidity and mortality, 23% chose that tuberculosis should no longer be a public health problem from 2050 onwards, and finally 16% felt that the incidence would fall below 1/million of population. The aim of the national tuberculosis control programme is to reduce morbidity and mortality due to tuberculosis. This objective is both social and epidemiological. [23] In fact, the national guide to tuberculosis control published in 2018 brings new missions:

• Ensure that all people suffering from tuberculosis have access to diagnosis and effective treatment in order to be cured;
• Breaking the chain of transmission of tuberculosis ;

• Reducing the social and economic burden of tuberculosis [24].

♲ The nurses participating in our study were aware of the general objective of the tuberculosis control programme. But this is not enough, as they need to learn more about the specific objectives.

XI. The role of nurses in the management of tuberculosis :

Our study showed that 87% of staff had treated patients with tuberculosis in various locations: pulmonary (52%), lymph node (29%), peritoneal (12%) and bone (1%).

♲ The majority of nurses dealt with the most frequent cases of tuberculosis, so the question arises: did they respect the protocols and universal rules for combating this endemic?

Analysis of the data collected shows that tuberculosis treatment at Gabès University Hospital begins in the emergency department, where nurses listed the following treatments: screening tests (44%), oxygen therapy (19%), peripheral venous access (27%) and monitoring of vital parameters (saturation, BP, temperature, etc.) (10%). Then there is hospitalisation in the two departments of pneumology and infectious diseases, where they request screening tests (16%), administration of treatment (50%), isolation (7%), compliance with treatment (10%) and monitoring of general condition (2%).Although the WHO emphasises the moral dimension by defining health as "A state of physical, mental and social well-being that does not consist solely in the absence of disease or infirmity."[25] The nurses in our study focused on the physical side of patient health, while neglecting the psychological and emotional aspects by providing care aimed solely at ridding the patient's body of germs. In addition, nurses in Japan specified that their support for patients should be empathetic, reliable, motivating and culturally appropriate, and that they should help the patient develop the basis for a healthier life after treatment. [26]

✑ This has led us to emphasise that in developed countries, the management of illness is not limited solely to the physical aspects of the disease, but also encompasses the social, mental and emotional aspects of the sick person. The patient's dignity must be respected throughout the treatment process, and the effects of the illness on his or her mental health are also considered and treated. This shows the great importance attached to the quality of healthcare in developed countries.

Among the results found in our study, 44% of the population studied were dissatisfied with care due to lack of resources (equipment, isolation rooms), work overload, psychological pressure, poor medical diagnosis and lack of moral support and respect. Among our staff, only 37% consider that care is satisfactory in relation to the resources available. However, 17% considered it to be good because it followed the protocol of the national tuberculosis programme, and 2% considered it to be excellent because the patients were satisfied.

To better assess the effectiveness of tuberculosis management, the World Health Organization states that the success rate of treatmentis estimated to be 90% in Tunisia in 2019 [27].These findingsat odds with the results of a retrospective descriptive and analytical study conducted in Morocco between 2015 and 2019. This study showed that cure was declared in more than a third of tuberculosis patients (35.12%) and that completion of treatment was also noted in more than a third of patients (37.48%). Lost to follow-up and deaths accounted for 15.59% and 2.76% of cases respectively. Therapeutic failure was noted in 0.63% of cases. [28]

✑ These figures show that treatment in Morocco is unsatisfactory, given the low cure rate and the appearance of side effects. In Tunisia, on the other hand, care is satisfactory despite the shortcomings and obstacles encountered (work overload, lack of resources, etc.). It is important to understand that the management of any disease can vary from one country to another due to many factors such as the situation of the country at the time, the health system, the resources available, the training of health professionals and also public awareness.

A recent survey carried out by the National Institute of Statistics showed that, on average, 54% of citizens were dissatisfied with the care provided in health centres, with a dissatisfaction rate of 79% in the South-West and 42% in the Centre-East. The reasons are linked to the lack of medicines, waiting times and the unavailability of medical staff. A proportion of 41% of citizens reported waiting times that were too long for a necessary operation, and almost 40% reported a lack of respect on the part of healthcare staff. [29] Measures need to be taken to improve the quality of care and guarantee patients access to better and more efficient care. To this end, the nurses in our survey suggested equipping the hospital with all the equipment needed for complementary examinations and screening (39%), health education (28%), compliance with the tuberculosis control protocol (12%), ongoing staff training (8%), good nutrition for patients (8%) and, last but not least, the importance of moral support (5%).

XII. Assessment of nursing knowledge of tuberculosis :

Theoretically, although the score attributed to this part is considered acceptable (16.5/28), the healthcare workers participating in our study do not have sufficient information concerning the evolution of this disease (chronicity, and stages), the types, the different locations, certain modes of transmission, and the institution to which they report. They also feel that their role is limited to administering the treatment, without researching the indications, counter-indications and possible side-effects. It is important for nurses to receive training and have their knowledge regularly updated if they are to offer quality care to patients with tuberculosis.

In practice, the management of tuberculosis by nurses can be approved (4/6) by rapid screening of new cases of tuberculosis in an emergency, regular monitoring of treatment, compliance with hygiene and prevention rules (wearing of bibs, isolation, hand washing and disinfection of equipment and patients' rooms). However, the care to be provided lacks active communication and moral support, which are important in all types of healthcare. They are particularly important in the management of tuberculosis, as the duration of treatment is often long and difficult, and patients can be stigmatised because of the disease. It is essential that healthcare professionals provide emotional support and effective communication to TB patients to help them manage their illness and maintain their quality of life.In this sense, a cross-sectional study using a self-questionnaire randomly administered to paramedical staff at the CHU la Rabta in Tunis. The survey was carried out between December 2015 and January 2016 and showed that overall scores were low with an average of 11.7 out of 21. The proportions The average number of correct answers in the areas of tuberculosis transmission, diagnosis and treatment, and NTP was 72.2%. However, better knowledge of the NTP was only associated with working in a pneumology or infectious diseases department.A number of gaps in the knowledge of healthcare staff have been identified, particularly in the diagnosis and treatment of the disease. Their level of knowledge should therefore be improved through ongoing professional training. [28] We found that the results of our research and those of the study carried out at the Rabta University Hospital showed a slight difference between the overall scores of our survey (20.5/34) and those of the other study (11.7/21). This can be explained by the fact that we worked in departments specialising in the management of tuberculosis (pneumology, infectious diseases and emergency departments). However, they included all the staff at Rabta Hospital. One point in common between the two studies was the need for continuous training, which provides nurses with a means of acquiring new skills and knowledge, enabling them to meet the needs of the population and patients. It also enables them to adapt to new working environments and take on new professional challenges.

RECOMMENDATION

At the end of our study, we put forward a number of recommendations aimed at optimising care and improving nurses' planning and knowledge:

- Plan the necessary material and human resources.

- Carrying out awareness-raising activities in hospitals nationwide to convey to healthcare staff the importance of ongoing training to improve care.
- Strict compliance with hospital hygiene rules through the implementation of specific and regular monitoring of services.
- It is vital to provide patients with clear, comprehensible information about their illness, the course of their treatment and how it will be monitored.
- Teamwork, which helps to promote active listening between patients and healthcare staff.
- Establishing and strengthening collaboration between the healthcare team to ensure correct diagnosis and appropriate management of the disease.
- When faced with any signs of tuberculosis, the patient should consult a facility capable of making the diagnosis and treating the patient.

CONCLUSION

According to the World Health Organisation (2023), tuberculosis is the thirteenth leading cause of death worldwide and the second leading cause of death from infectious diseases. It is mainly found in low- and middle-income countries. According to estimates, 10.6 million people will have developed tuberculosis worldwide and 1.6 million will die from the disease in 2021. [30] As a result, good prevention and effective treatment are needed to eradicate this disease. This is what prompted us to choose this disease as the subject of our end-of-study project, all the more so as it is widespread and endemic in Tunisia. We conducted a descriptive, cross-sectional and analytical study of 60 nurses with the aim of assessing the quality of care and the role, skills and knowledge of nurses in the fight against this endemic. The results of our survey showed that the nurses' responses were somewhat general to what has been described in the literature as neglect, lack of continuing education and work overload. We found that carers need awareness-raising and appropriate training to enhance their theoretical and practical knowledge in order to achieve the objectives set by the national tuberculosis control programme, which is based on preventive care, essentially vaccination.

BIBLIOGRAPHY

[1] Wikipedia. (2022). History of tuberculosis. Spotted at https://fr.wikipedia.org/wiki/Histoire_de_la_tuberculose (Accessed on 15.05.2023)

[2] : Koné, Z., Daix Ahou, J., Samaké, K., Bakayoko-yéo, S., Coulibaly, G., Kouao Domoua Serge, M. (2019). Tuberculosis-HIV co-infection: state of Knowledge and attitudes of healthcare staff in pneumology settings in Abidjan. Abidjan, ivory coast. Retrieved from: https://www.revues-ufhb-ci.org/fichiers/FICHIR_ARTICLE_2611.pdf (Accessed on 15.05.2023)

[3] : the national tuberculosis management guide. (2018).Aetiology and pathogenesis of tuberculosis. Retrieved from: http://www.santetunisie.rns.tn/images/docs/anis/actualite/2018/octobre/3010201 8Guide-PNLT-2018.pdf (consulted on 16.05.2023)

[4] : Tudor, C. (2019, March).course-pneumology-tuberculosis. Infirmier.com Spotted àhttps://www.infirmiers.com/etudiants/cours-et-tests/cours- pneumology-tuberculosis#:~:text=The%20nurses%20are%20in%20first%C3%A8re,a%2Dt%2Delle%20d%C3%A9clar%C3%A9. (Consulted on 15.05.2023)

[5] World Health Organization. (2023). World tuberculosis control report: incidence of tuberculosis. Geneva, Switzerland: World Bank Group. Available at :https://donnees.banquemondiale.org/indicator/SH.TBS.INCD?locations=TN (Accessed on 16.05.2023)

[6] Maddeh, S., Mouelhi, D., Jlaiel, N., jdidi, M. T, Khraifi, M., Oueslati, B., Aouadi, S. (2022). Revue des maladies respiratoires actualités : profil épidémiologique de la tuberculose dans la région du nord de la Tunisie, 14,157-. 158. Retrieved from: https://doi.org/10.1016/j.rmra.2021.11.257 (Accessed on 19.05.2023)

[7] Marrakchi, C., Maàlouli, l., Lahiani, D., Hammami, B., Boudawara, T., Zribi, M., & Ben jemaa, M. (2010). Médicine et maladie infectieuses : diagnostic de la tuberculose ganglionnaire périphérique en Tunisie, 40,119 /122. Retrieved from :

https://doi.org/10.1016/j.medmal.2009.10.014 (consulted on 20.05.2023)

[8] : Hamzaoui, G., Amro, L., Sajiai, H., Serhane, H., Moumen, N., Ennezari, A., & yazidi, A.(2014). Lymph node tuberculosis: epidemiological and

therapeutic aspects, about 357 cases. Retrieved from:

https://www.ncbi.nlm.nih.gov/pmc/articles/PMC4345207/(Accessed on 20.05.2023)

[9] Elbarni, R., Lahkim, M., & Achour, A. (2012). Abdominal pseudotumor tuberculosis. Retrieved from:

https://www.ncbi.nlm.nih.gov/pmc/articles/PMC3542810/#:~:text=The%20tuber culosis%20abdominal%20pseudo%2Dtumour%2C%20rare%20m%C3%AAm e%20in%20countries%20d,still%20in%20cases%20of%20complication. (Accessed on 20.05.2023)

[10] : Doudo, T., Yeo Gningniminni, D., Coulibaly, B., Bla Claire, K., Kara Gérard, L., Koffi Sosthéne, K., ... Tra Goin Lou Tina, V. (2012).Étude des connaissances, attitudes et pratiques sur la tuberculose dans les 19 anciennes régions sanitaires de Cote d'ivoire. University of Bouake, cote d'ivoire.

https://allianceciv.org/alliance/pdf/ENQUETE_CAP_TB_2012_RAPPORT_FI NAL.pdf

[11] Edward, A. (2022). Tuberculosis (TB). Retrieved from: https://www.msdmanuals.com/fr/professional/maladies-infectious/mycobact%C3%A9ria/tuberculosis-tb (consulted on 20.05.2023)

[12] Cisse, A. (2009). Aspects épidémiologiques et cliniques de la tuberculose chez les enfants de 0-15 ans dans les six centres de sante de référence de Bamako (Doctoral thesis). University of Bamako, Mali.

https://www.keneya.net/fmpos/theses/2009/med/pdf/09M120.pdf (consulted on 20.05.2023)

[13] Aazri, L., Aitbatahar, s., Amro, L. (2020). Journal of respiratory diseases news: risk factors and diagnosis of tuberculosis, 12,264. Retrieved from:

https://www.sciencedirect.com/science/article/abs/pii/S187712031937288 (consulted on 21.05.2023)

[14] Respiratory Fund. (2023). What are the screening tests for tuberculosis? Retrieved from :

https://fares.be/tuberculose/f-a-q/quels-sont-les-tests-de-depistage-de-la-tuberculose (consulted on 21.05.2023)

[15] :, N. Bouhedda,. Lellou,(2018).Review of Respiratory Diseases: Living

with sequelae of tuberculosis, 35, A181. Retrieved from:

https://www.em-consulte.com/article/1194885/vivre-avec-des-sequelles-de-tuberculose (consulted on 21.05.2023)

[16] Institut Pasteur. (2021). Tuberculosis. Retrieved from:
https://www.pasteur.fr/fr/centre-medical/fiches-maladies/tuberculose#traitement (consulted on 21.05.2023)

[17] : Critchley, J., Orton, L., Pearson, F. (2014). Adjuvant corticosteroid therapy in pulmonary tuberculosis. Available at:

https://www.cochranelibrary.com/cdsr/doi/10.1002/14651858.CD011370/full/fr (consulté le 21.05.2023)

[18] Nathan, C. (2015). Anti inflammatory. Retrieved from:
https://www.allodocteurs.fr/maladies-maladies-infectieuses-et-tropicales-tuberculosis-an-anti-inflammatory-8082.html (consulted on 21.05.2023)

[19] Libbey, J. (2010). L'essentiel de l'information scientifique et médicale, 20.89. Retrieved from:

.https://www.onmne.tn/wp- content/uploads/2020/10/tuberculosis_fighting_5.pdf

(Accessed on 22.05.2023)
[20] : the national tuberculosis management guide (2018).BCG. Retrieved from:

http://www.santetunisie.rns.tn/images/docs/anis/actualite/2018/octobre/3010201 8Guide-PNLT-2018.pdf (Accessed on 22.05.2023)

[21] Fonds des affections respiratoire asbl (2013). Contagiousness and isolation. Retrieved from:

https://www.fares.be/tuberculose/infos-pour-professionnels/tuberculose-disease/contagiosis-and-isolation (Consulted on 22.05.2023)

[22] National tuberculosis control programme (2010). The Notifiable Communicable Diseases (NCD) System - Retrieved from :

https://www.ccmtunisie.org.tn/wp-content/uploads/2017/02/plannationalse.pdf (Accessed on 25.05.2023)

[23] National Tuberculosis Control Programme (2010). Monitoring and evaluation system objective. Retrieved from:https://www.ccmtunisie.org.tn/wp-

content/uploads/2017/02/plannationalse.pdf (Accessed on 25.05.2023)

[24] National tuberculosis management guide (2018). Mission. Retrieved from:

http://www.santetunisie.rns.tn/images/docs/anis/actualite/2018/octobre/3010201
8Guide-PNLT-2018.pdf (Accessed on 25.05.2023)

[25] World Health Organisation. (1946). Preamble to the Constitution of the
World Health Organization, as adopted by the International Health Conference.
Available at

https://www.who.int/fr/about/frequently-asked-
questions#:~:text=How%20the%20WHO%20does%C3%A9define%2Delle,disea
se%2 0or%20disease%C3%A9%C2%BB. (Accessed on 25.05.2023)

[26] World Health Organization. (Communicable diseases: tuberculosis.

[27] World Health Organization. (2023). Tuberculosis treatment success rate:
incidence of tuberculosis. Geneva, Switzerland: World Bank Group. Available
on :

https://donnees.banquemondiale.org/indicator/SH.TBS.INCD?locations=TN
(Accessed on 16.05.2023)

[28] Belhadj, H., Belhaj Yahia, M., El Abassi, A., Sabri, B. (2016). Le droit a la
santé en Tunisie (report on the right to health in Tunisia).association tunisienne
de défense du droit a la santé, Tunisia. Retrieved from:
https://ftdes.net/rapports/ATDDS.pdf (Accessed on 25.05.2023)
[29] World Health Organization. (2023). Tuberculosis. Retrieved from:
https://**www.who.int/fr/news-room/fact-sheets/detail/tuberculosis** (Accessed
on 26.05.2023)

APPENDIX

Questionnaire

We are Hasnaoui Khadija and Bourassi Nesrine, 3rd year students at the Higher Institute of Nursing Sciences in Gabès.

As part of our end-of-study project, we will be submitting a questionnaire to you in order to refine my research:

A.Socio-demographic and professional characteristics :

1. You are a : A man A woman

2. How old are you?

-30 years 31 to 40 years 41 to 50 years+50 years

1. How long have you worked in the hospital?

Less than 5 years 10 years11 - 15 years over 15 years

2. Which department do you belong to?

3. Work period :

Morning afternoon night

B. Knowledge study :

I. The definition of tuberculosis :

1. Do you have any ideas about tuberculosis? Yes No

2. How is tuberculosis defined?
 Is a chronic progressive infection with a latent phase and possibly an active phase
 Is an infectious disease caused by a mycobacterium, Mycobacterium tuberculosis, which most often affects the lungs but can also affect other organs.
 Contagious disease caused by the koch bacillus and certain external causes (malnutrition, lack of sunlight, etc.).

II. Participation in a training course on tuberculosis :

1. Do you attend any training courses on tuberculosis?
Yes no

III. The epidemiology of tuberculosis :

1. According to you, the latest statistics on tuberculosis will be carried out in
2021: How many cases declared in Tunisia in this year?

20 new cases/100,000 36 new cases/100,000
35 new cases/100,000 34 new cases/100,000

2. The incidence of tuberculosis in the Gabès region :
ignificantly lower than the national average Close to the national average
Higher than the national average

IV. The different types of tuberculosis :

1. What are the most common types of tuberculosis according to location?
Lung bone lymph node peritoneal neuro-meningeal skin multiple locations
other
1. adenopathies in lymph node tuberculosis are located in the: cervical
mediastinal subclavicular axillary
2. Which of the following organs may be affected by tuberculosis?
peritoneal :
The omentum intestinal tract liver spleen Parietal and visceral peritoneum
genitals

V. Clinical signs of tuberculosis :

1. Tick the symptoms of tuberculosis :

Vomiting fever anorexiafatigue Persistent cough for more than two weeks
haemoptysisWeight loss Night sweats infectious syndrome

AdenopathyDiarrhoea   Joint pain

VI. Etiopathogenesis :

1. Tuberculosis:

- Is it a disease :

- Parasitic Viral Bacterial
1. What germ causes the disease?
 Microbacteium tuberculosis (BK)
 Streptococcus pyogenes Staphylococcus aureus
2. Are there other reservoirs of tuberculosis than humans?
Yes no
3. In your opinion, what is the mode of transmission of tuberculosis (pulmonary and extra-pulmonary)?
Air Transplacental Blood Orofaecal
4. Pulmonary tuberculosis is a disease that is transmitted by :
Airborne Transplacental Blood Orofaecal
5. Extra-pulmonary tuberculosis is usually due to the haematogenous dissemination of pulmonary tuberculosis:
 Yes no
6. What are the stages of tuberculosis?
And organise them in chronological order.
 Primary infection active infection latent infection
1. What are the risk factors for tuberculosis?
Promiscuity malnutrition children under 5 years of age
Elderly Diabetic Immune deficiency Poor socio-economic conditions Vitamin D deficiency Lack of BCG vaccination Drug and tobacco use

Screening tests :

1. What tests are needed to screen for tuberculosis? IDR
 Testing for BK in sputum Testing for BK in urine

Gamma interferon release test Other
Which one if other

VII. Potential complications of tuberculosis :

1. Tuberculosis can have certain complications.

Caverns respiratory failure arteritis and osteitis pulmonary embolism occlusion fistula

Superinfection Spread to other sites

VIII. Tuberculosis treatments :

1. tuberculosis can be treated with :

Anti-inflammatories Antibiotics

Tuberculosis drugs Corticosteroids

Antifungals chemotherapy

2. Is the treatment made available to patients free of charge by the Ministry of Health?Yes no

IX. Preventive measures :

1. BCG vaccination: This is a live vaccine.
The vial of vaccine contains at least 10 doses
The vaccine is to be given as a strict intradermal injection All newborns must be vaccinated.
Indicated for pregnant women and immunocompromised patients
2. Is isolation necessary for all types of tuberculosis? Yes no
3. Does the patient require isolation for pulmonary tuberculosis? Yes no
If not, what do you do?
4. Do you often wear a bib when administering treatment to a patient?Yes no
5. Is tuberculosis a notifiable disease? Yes no
If yes, to whom do you declare?
6. Why is it necessary to carry out a health survey of the people around a patient?
7.what are the objectives of the national tuberculosis programme?
By 2050, tuberculosis will no longer be a public health problem.Incidence will be less than 1 per million inhabitants.
Reducing morbidity and mortality

X. the nursing role in the management of tuberculosis :

1. Have you ever been in contact with patients suffering from tuberculosis of any kind? Yes no
Location of tuberculosis:
What should you do?
Emergency:
During hospitalisation:
How would you rate the way patients with tuberculosis are treated in your department?
Unsatisfactory Acceptable/satisfactory
Good Excellent
Explain
2. What proposals do you have for improving the care of patients with tuberculosis in your department?

Thank you for your participation

SUMMARY

Introduction: Tuberculosis is considered to be a global public health concern due to its increasing incidence and as a major cause of morbidity and mortality in many countries, particularly in the developing world.

Objectives: The aim of this study was to assess the knowledge of healthcare workers about tuberculosis in order to identify any lack of knowledge about the management of tuberculosis patients in the governorate of Gabès.

Materials and methods: This is a descriptive, cross-sectional study of 60 nurses at Gabès University Hospital in the Pneumology, Infectious Diseases and Emergency Department, using an anonymous questionnaire. The data were collected and analysed over a 3-month period in February, March and April 2023.

Results: Our population consisted of 60 nurses, the majority of whom were women with less than 5 years' professional experience. Only 32% of the participants had attended previous training courses on this disease. In addition, 87% of the nurses had already treated patients with tuberculosis. We found that a minority of nursing staff knew that BCG vaccination is recommended for newborns and that it must be administered intradermally. Most of those surveyed (44%) were dissatisfied with the quality of care in their departments because of the difficulties encountered (lack of resources, work overload, etc.). They emphasised two key aspects for improving tuberculosis management: providing the hospital with all the equipment needed to carry out complementary examinations and screening (39%) and providing regular health education (28%). Based on our results, we concluded that the general level of nurses' theoretical and practical knowledge of tuberculosis is acceptable.

Conclusion: Prevention is the most important pillar in reducing the contamination, transmission and morbidity and mortality associated with tuberculosis. Healthcare workers therefore need to be made aware of the problem and receive ongoing training to enhance their theoretical and practical knowledge in order to defeat this scourge and achieve the objectives set by the national tuberculosis control programme.

Key words: tuberculosis, knowledge, nurses, treatment, BK, BCG.

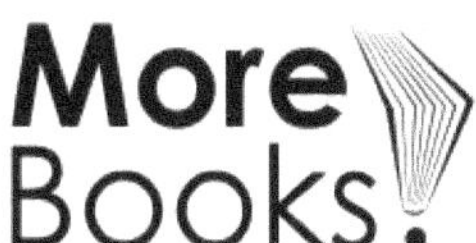

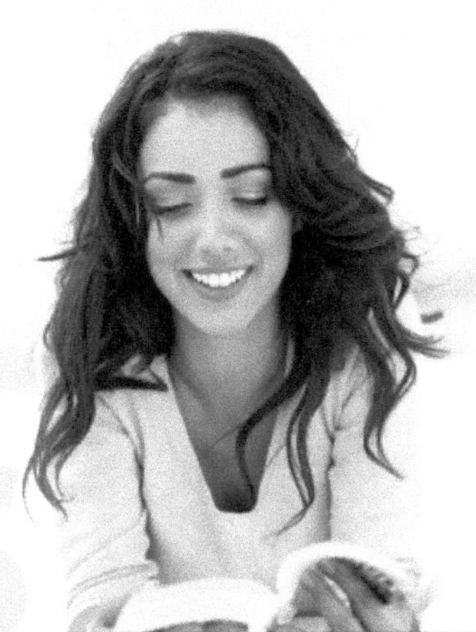

I want morebooks!

Buy your books fast and straightforward online - at one of world's fastest growing online book stores! Environmentally sound due to Print-on-Demand technologies.

Buy your books online at
www.morebooks.shop

Kaufen Sie Ihre Bücher schnell und unkompliziert online – auf einer der am schnellsten wachsenden Buchhandelsplattformen weltweit! Dank Print-On-Demand umwelt- und ressourcenschonend produziert.

Bücher schneller online kaufen
www.morebooks.shop

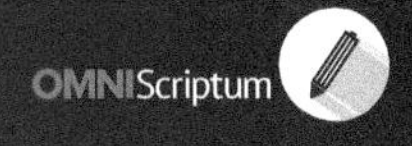

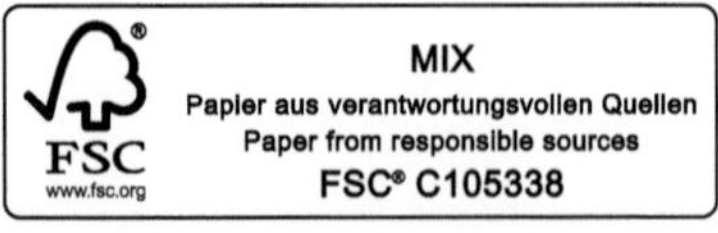
MIX
Papier aus verantwortungsvollen Quellen
Paper from responsible sources
FSC® C105338
FSC
www.fsc.org

Printed by Books on Demand GmbH, Norderstedt / Germany